I0101590

Yoga

To Beat

Depression

and Anxiety

Monique Joiner Siedlak

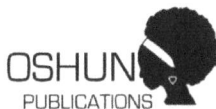

OSHUN
PUBLICATIONS

Printed in the United States of America

Second Edition 2018

ISBN-13: 978-1-948834-46-9

Publisher
www.oshunpublications.com

Disclaimer
All the material contained in this book is provided for educational and informational purposes only. No responsibility can be taken for any results or outcomes resulting from the use of this material. While every attempt has been made to provide information that is both accurate and effective, the author does not assume any responsibility for the accuracy or use/misuse of this information.

Yoga Poses Photos

Pixabay.com

Freepik.com

Dreamstime.com

Cover Design by Monique Joiner Siedlak

Cover Image by Pixabay.com

Logo Design by Monique Joiner Siedlak

Logo Image by Pixabay.com

Sign up to email list: www.mojosiedlak.com

Other Books in the Series

Yoga for Beginners

Yoga for Stress

Yoga for Back Pain

Yoga for Weight Loss

Yoga for Flexibility

Yoga for Advanced Beginners

Yoga for Fitness

Yoga for Runners

Yoga for Energy

Yoga for Your Sex Life

Yoga for Menstruation

Table of Contents

Introduction

In this fast paced world, there is little time for an individual to sit and relax. And because we struggle so hard to keep up with our reputation and other people's expectations, we often overlook and disregard our own persisting feelings that demand something from us. One of those feelings is characterized by sadness, loneliness, and self-pity that all pile up under one roof to give shelter to an uninvited guest, depression.

Anxiety comes in many forms, disturbing those who suffer from its various forms, forms including generalized anxiety as well as acute anxiety disorder. Anxiety creates feelings of defeat, anger, panic, persistent fear, low self-esteem and limited control. People want to avoid anxiety. Yet for others it is a constant struggle, leading them to try medications to treat it, hoping to be released from its powerful clutches. Practicing yoga is a great way to take the challenge of anxiety head on, proactively subduing it effects.

Yoga is a great way to come to terms and target your depression by focusing absolutely on self-awareness with the attainment of peace. Inside these pages are yoga exercises to help you in to reducing your depression to past tense.

All these poses will help you cope with the jumbled up thoughts in your mind to pinpoint the source of your depression. Yoga will help your body, mind, and soul to work in unison and relax your nerves as well as various points in the body.

Depression will be a thing of the past, but before it does become your past, you need to face it head-on. Where there's a will there's a way, you do not have to continue feeling depressed when you can do something as simple and peaceful as yoga. Just think of depression as the sign that you haven't been taking care of yourself enough, and now that you've realized it, go ahead and begin your yoga routine today.

Cat Pose (Marjariasana)

The Cat Pose consists of relaxation of your back by taking on a posture of a cat. It is generally used to begin a yoga exercise, following the initial establishment of breath, by going through cat and cow pose. Amidst a nice steady foundation in tabletop, this movement allows us grounding as we begin to gently open up the back body and stimulate the core. It's most indispensable goal, though, is the opportunity it enables to combine the breath with activity.

How to Do

Start off by placing yourself in a tabletop position, using your hands and knees as the four legs of a table. Your knees would be positioned up and down below your hips. Your shoulders, wrists, and elbows should be parallel and perpendicular to the ground. You will then focus your eyes on the floor, with your head in a middle position.

Let your breath out and allow your spine to curve by directing it upward to the ceiling. Your shoulders and knees should be in the recommended four-legged position. At this moment, let your head somewhat fall towards the floor. Do not fall so far that your chin is pressed into the sternal hollow of your chest.

While inhaling, once again come back to the typical tabletop position. Maintain breathing in and breathing out deeply while transferring your position from relaxed to alert. Maintain until you feel the relaxation in your spine.

Benefits

The Cat Pose gradually works your spine as well as its muscles. It stretches your neck, back, and torso. In addition to improving the functions of your belly organs, it calms your mind by alleviating it from tension and stress.

Tips

The Cat Pose is an easy and simple yoga pose to relax your fatigued body. Ask your partner or friend to lay a hand in the middle of your shoulder blades if you are finding it challenging to bring a curve in the upper section of your back which will then result in a prompt triggering of that area.

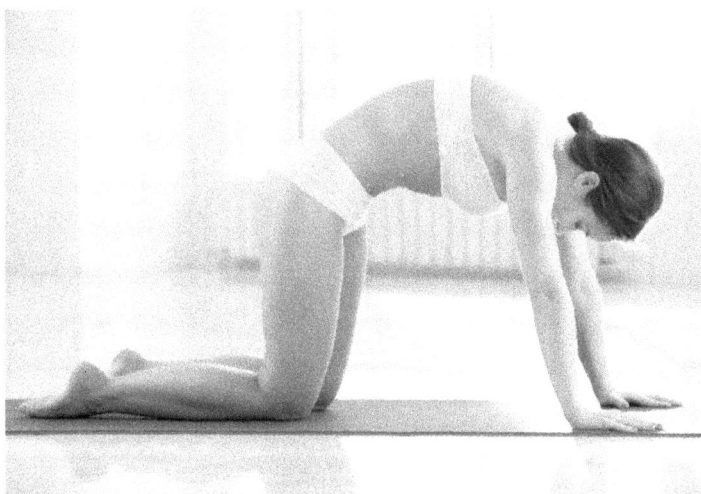

Cow Pose (Bitilasana)

The Cow Pose is regularly instructed in sequence with the Cat Pose to do a mild warm-up sequence. When practiced together, the poses help to stretch the body and prepare it for other activity.

You will inhale through the Cow Pose and exhale through the Cat Pose.

How to Do

Begin with your hands and knees in a tabletop position. You should make sure you align your shoulders above your wrists and your hips are aligned above your knees. Come to a horizontal back by lengthening the spine. Place your head and neck in a non-aligned position, staring down in the direction of the floor.

Breathe in and curve your back. Elevate through your glutes and the crown of your head and allow your belly to drop toward the floor. Rotate the shoulders up and down the back, feeling the back bend in your thoracic spine. Widen up your chest.

Hold the Cow Pose for one breath. Exhale and come back to a nonaligned, tabletop position again. You can also practice this in combination with the Cat Pose, alternating inhales with the Cow Pose and exhales with the Cat Pose.

Benefits

This is a gentle backbend that works with the Cat Pose to awaken the spine. Opens the chest, shoulders and upper back. Teaches the connection between inhaling and expanding and exhaling and contracting.

Tip

Care for your neck by widening your shoulder blades and pulling your shoulders down, away from your ears.

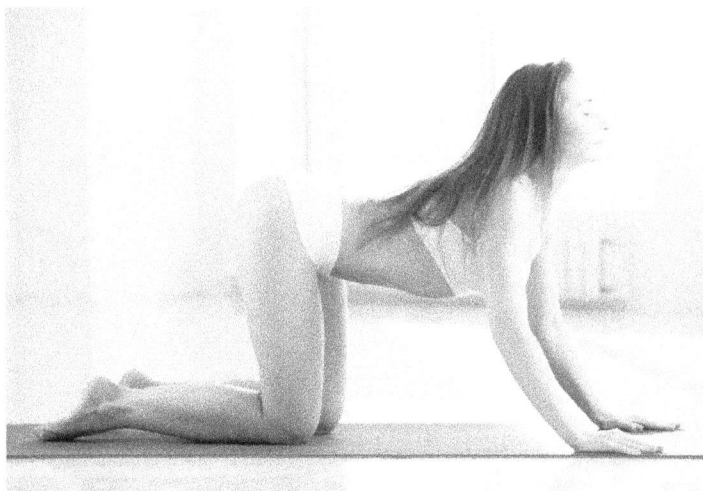

Bridge Pose (Setu Bandha Sarvangasana)

The Bridge Pose is a beginning backbend that helps to open your chest and stretch your thighs.

How to Do

To begin, lie supine (on your back). Fold your knees and keep your feet hip distance apart on the floor, ten to twelve inches from your pelvis, with your knees and ankles in a straight line. With your arms beside your body, place your palms faced down.

Breathe in, while slowly lifting your lower back, middle back and upper back off the floor. Gently roll in your shoulders. Touch your chest to your chin without bringing the chin down. Support your weight with your shoulders, arms, and feet. Feel your buttocks firm up in this pose. Both your thighs should be parallel to each other and to the floor.

You could interlock your fingers and push your hands on the floor to lift your torso a bit more up if you want or you could support your back with your palms. Keep breathing easily.

Hold this pose for a minute or two and then exhale as you gently release the pose.

Benefits

The Bridge Pose strengthens your back, opens the chest, and improves your spinal mobility.

Tips

After you roll your shoulders under, be sure not to pull them away from your ears. This often overstrains your neck. Raise the tops of your shoulders toward your ears and push your inner shoulder blades away from your spine.

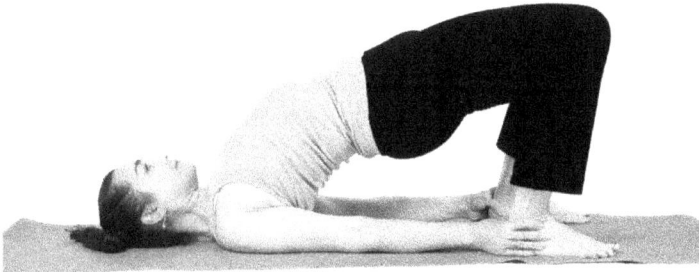

Fish Pose (Matsyasana)

The Fish Pose is performed often as a counterbalance poses to the Shoulder Stand Pose. It stretches your upper body in the opposite way. The Fish Pose has a lot of possibilities because it encourages the throat and crown.

How to Do

Begin by lying on your back. Keeping your feet are together, relax your hands at the side of the body. Inhale. With palms facing down, place the hands underneath your hips. Draw your elbows close to each other and exhale.

Elevate your head and chest, and then inhale. You should extend your legs with your head relaxed back, without adding pressure on your head.

Keeping the chest elevated, lower the head backward and touch the top of your head to the floor. Exhale; allow the chest to open finding awareness of relaxed backbend.

Hold this pose for as long as you can while taking soothing long breaths in and out. With each exhalation, relax in the pose. Raise your head, while lowering your chest and head to the floor. Bring your hands back along the sides of your body and relax.

Benefits

The Fish Pose can help headaches caused by stiffness of the neck. It relaxes Spinal Cord and back muscle tissues. It aids in relieving asthma and respiratory disorders. This yoga pose, when practiced regularly, helps to remedy impotence. Also eases anxiety, mild backache, fatigue and menstrual pain.

Tips

If your head does not comfortably come to the floor, position a blanket or block under your head or slightly lower your chest.

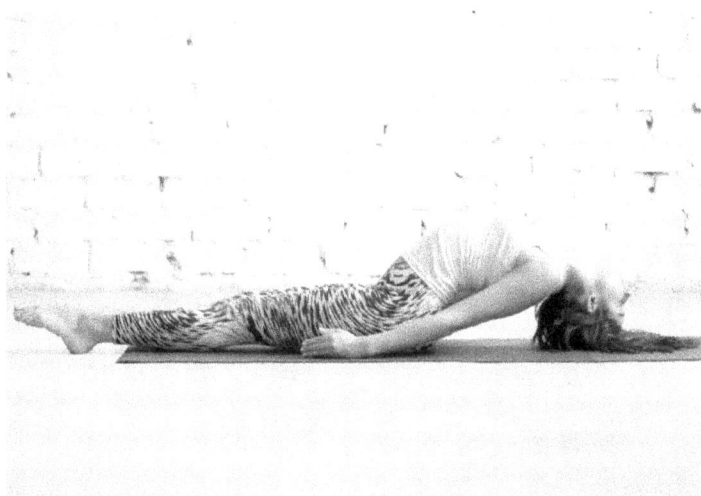

Cobra Pose (Bhujangasana)

The Cobra Pose is a familiar Yoga backbend. When you perform the Cobra Pose, you stretch the front of your torso and spine.

How to Do

Lie face down on the floor. Extend your legs back, with the tops of your feet on the floor. Stretch your hands on the floor beneath your shoulders. Squeeze the elbows back into your body. Push the tops of your feet, thighs, and pubis powerfully into the floor.

On an inhalation, start to straighten your arms to raise your chest off the floor. Go only to a height at which you can sustain a connection throughout your pubis to your legs. Press your tailbone toward the pubis and raise the pubis toward your navel. Narrow the hip, compressing but don't harden your buttocks.

Firm the shoulder blades against the back, puffing the side ribs forward. Lift through the top of the sternum but avoid pushing the front ribs forward, which only hardens the lower back. Distribute the backbend evenly throughout the full spine.

Hold the pose anywhere from fifteen to thirty seconds, breathing freely. Release back to the floor with an exhalation.

Benefits

The Cobra Pose is best known for its capability to build up the flexibility of your spine. It stretches the chest along with strengthening your spine and shoulders. It further assists in opening the lungs and stimulating the abdominal organs, improving digestion.

An energizing backbend, the Cobra Pose can reduce stress and fatigue. It also firms and tones the shoulders, abdomen, and buttocks, and assists in easing back pain.

Tips

The Cobra Pose will be able to energize and warm up the body, getting it ready for the deeper backbends in your yoga routine.

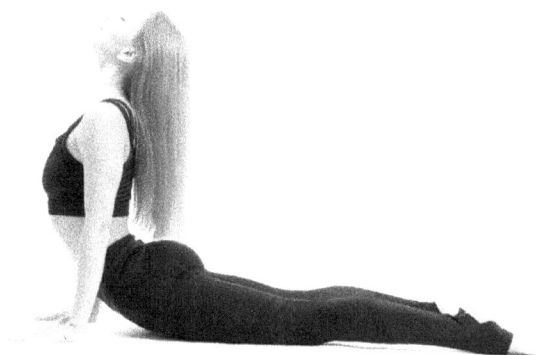

Plow Pose (Halasana)

The Plow Pose prepares the sphere of your body and mind for a deep transformation.

How to Do

Lie on your backside and bend your legs. While keeping your legs together, set your feet on the floor. Raise your feet and pelvis from the floor. You can assist with your hands, and lower your knees onto your forehead. You can then press your palms against your back or clasp your hands and lower them on the floor behind your back. Go back, rolling your spine back on the floor to release.

Benefits

The Plow Pose opens your neck, shoulders, and back. By compressing your abdomen, it massages and tones your digestive organs, which increases your body's cleansing. This pose promotes and regulates your thyroid gland, helps get rid of excess mucus and phlegm, and regulates your breath.

Tip

With this pose, you may have an inclination to overtax your neck by straining your shoulders too far away from your ears. As the tops of your shoulders should push down into the support, they should be raised toward the ears to keep the back of your neck and throat soft. Open your sternum by compressing the shoulder blades against your back.

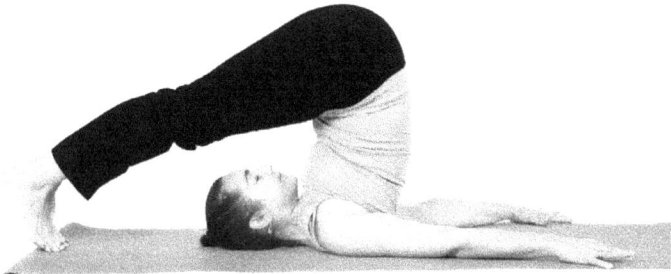

Head-To-Knee Forward Bend Pose (Janu Sirsasana)

The Head-to-Knee Forward Bend Pose is a deep, forward bend that soothes the mind and releases stress. It is frequently practiced near the end of a sequence, when the body is warm, to set up the body for even deeper forward bends.

How to Do

Start in a seated pose with your legs stretched. Bend the right leg, pulling the bottom of the foot to the upper inside of the right thigh. The right knee must rest steadily on the floor. Take both hands to both sides of the left leg. Breathe in and turn towards your extended leg. Breathe out and fold forward. Exhale slowly and deeply for three to five breaths. To come out of the pose, breathe in back to the beginning position. Repeat the other side.

Benefits

Helps tone your legs and burn the fats in your abdominal.

Tip

You can sit up on a blanket if your hips are tight. Place a strap about the extended foot, If you like or hold an end of the strap in each hand as you forward bend.

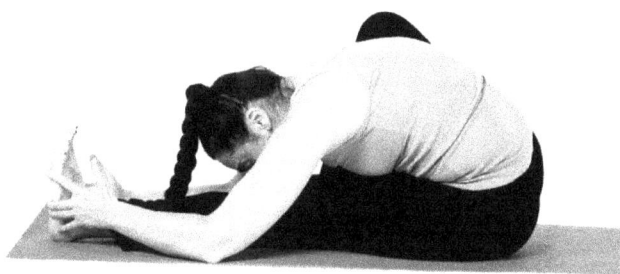

Warrior One Pose (Virabhadrasana)

The Warrior One Pose is the first of a series of three and is a focusing and strengthening pose, aimed to build a link, grounding you with the Earth's energy.

How to Do

Move your right foot toward the back of your mat to come into Warrior I. Bring your right heel to the floor and turn your right toes out to about a forty-five-degree angle. Bend your left knee over the left ankle. You might need to correct the length of your stance from the front to back. You can also broaden your stance from side to side for a greater stability. Maintain the position of your hips that same as it was in Mountain pose, with the hips pointing forward.

While breathing in, bring your arms up over your head. Your arm position may vary in relation to the flexibility in your shoulders. The typical position is with the palms touching above, but you may decide on keeping your palms apart at shoulder distance or you can bend at your elbows and open your arms resembling a saguaro cactus. A slight backbend will open the heart and the gaze move toward the fingertips.

Benefits

The Warrior One Pose helps strengthen and tone your arms, legs and lower back. It also helps increase stamina and improves the balance in your body.

Tips

Warrior One Pose has been shown with the heel of your front foot aligned with the arch of your back foot as if you were on a balance beam. This division enables the hips to square more.

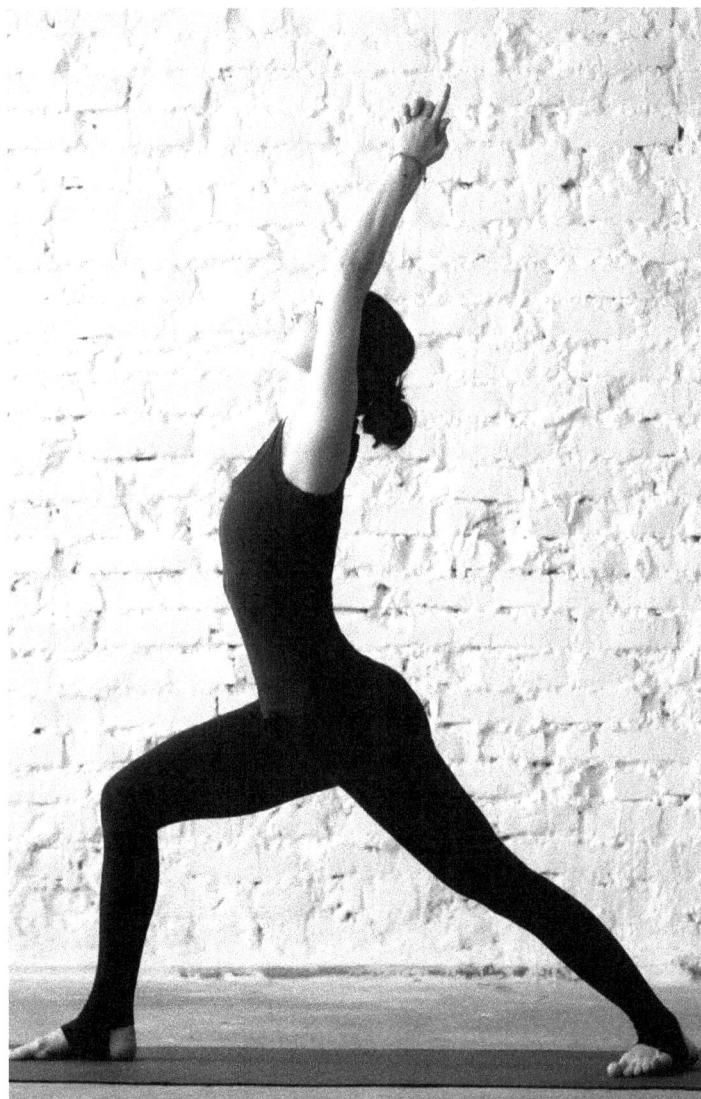

Warrior Two Pose (Virabhadrasana II)

The Warrior Two Pose is the second of a sequence of three yoga poses that improve strength and stamina.

How to Do

From the Downward Facing Dog, step your left foot to the inside your left hand. Bend your left knee over your ankle so your thigh is parallel to the floor. Swivel on the ball of your right foot to bring your right heel to your mat. Your right foot should be at a 90-degree angle with the sole planted.

Your front heel is lined up with your back arch. Rise to stand. Open your hips to the right side of your mat. Your torso will face right. Extend your left arm toward the front of the mat and your right arm toward the back of the mat with your palms facing down. Keep both arms parallel to the floor. Release your shoulders away from your ears. Reach out through the fingertips of both hands.

Turn your head to face the front of your mat. Your gaze is forward over the left hand. Both thighs are rotating outward.

Engage your triceps to support your arms, your quadriceps to support your legs, and your belly to support your torso.

After several breaths, windmill your hands down to either side of your left foot and step back to Downward Dog. Stay here for a few breaths or go through a transition before repeating the pose with the right foot forward.

Benefits

Tones the abdomen, strengthen your legs and arms and opens your chest and shoulders.

Tips

When you bend the right knee to a right angle, bend it with a meaningful exhalation, and point the inside the right knee in the direction of the little-toe side of the right foot.

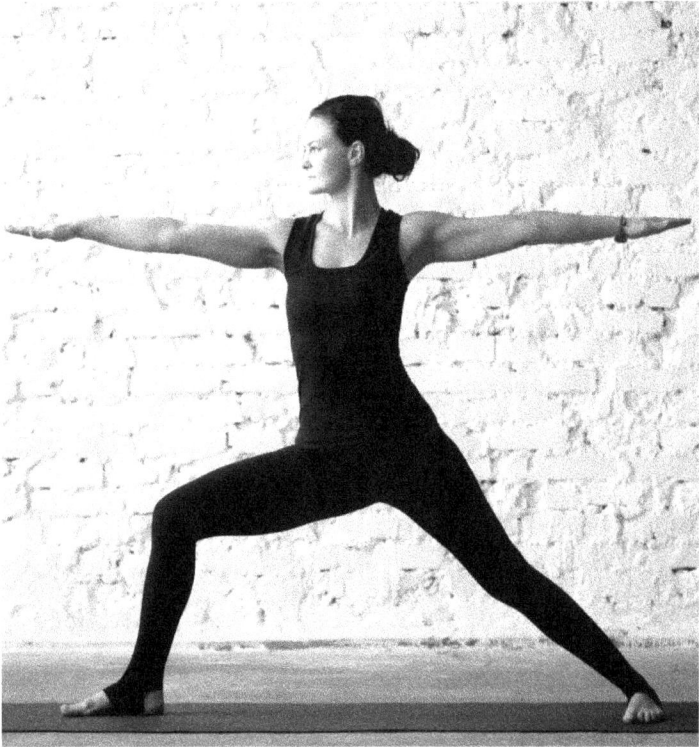

Reverse Warrior Pose (Viparita Virabhadrasana)

The Reverse Warrior Pose is a standing yoga pose which stretches the waist and energizes the entire body. It's usually practiced as part of a Dancing Warrior sequence which moves from Warrior One to Warrior Two and then straight into Reverse Warrior.

How to Do

Begin in Warrior Two Pose. Bring your back hand down to your rear leg, with the palm facing down. Turn the front hand, palm facing up towards the ceiling. Breathe in, extend your front arm up towards the ceiling, palm facing towards the back of the room. Keeping your hips open as you would in Warrior Two Pose, reach your heart up towards the sky. Continue to bend deeply into your front knee; while trying to keep your weight equally distributed on your front foot. Take breaths here for up to thirty seconds, and then return to Warrior Two Pose.

Benefits

The Reverse Warrior Pose strengthens your legs, improves balance, opens the side body, improves spinal mobility, and your core strength.

Tips

It is important that you stay focused on the various points of alignment. Work on getting your leg and feet positioning first. Allow the pose be developed from the floor upwards. Make certain that your front knee stays aligned with the ankle that is in front. Avoid allowing the knee from wandering to the inside. This can trigger a strain in the joint of the knees. Your front shin should be kept vertical. Buildup your stance as needed to make certain that your knees do not move in front past your ankle. You should as well keep in mind that it is not necessary for you to go too far in the backbend. If you feel a collapse or crunching in your lower back get out of the backbend immediately to regain the space in the spine.

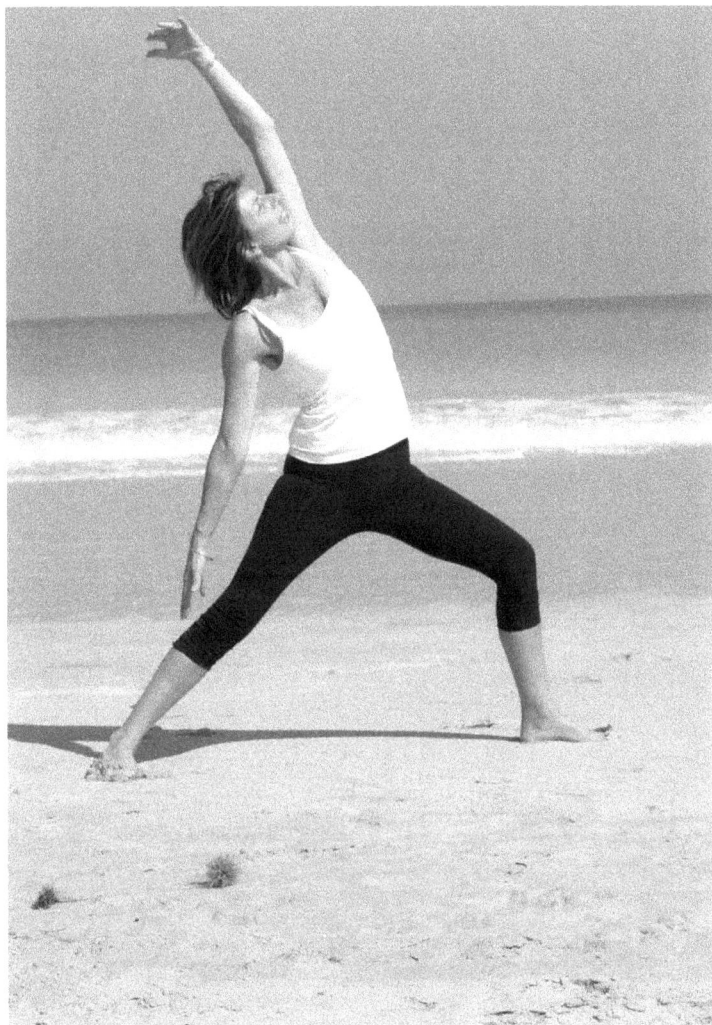

Standing Forward Fold Pose (Uttanasana)

Standing Forward Fold Pose is an important component of the Sun Salutations. This pose is used to train the body for deeper forward bends.

How to Do

Begin by Standing with your feet together. Bend your knees somewhat and bend your torso, not the lower back, over your legs, shift from your hips. Put your hands on the floor in front of you or next to your feet.

Breathe in and expand your chest to elongate your spine. Keep your focus fixed forward.

Breathe out and press both legs straight. Raise your kneecaps and twist your upper and inner thighs back. Without hyperextending, maintain your legs straight.

Extend your torso down without rounding your back, on an exhalation. Stay long through your neck, lengthening the top of your head toward the ground. Pull your shoulders down your back.

Benefits

The Standing Forward Fold pose extends your spinal column and stretches the back muscles as well as the backs of your legs.

Tip

Bend your knees to increase the stretch in the backs of your legs. Take care not to straighten the knees by locking them back; as an alternative, allow them to straighten as the two ends of each leg move farther spaced out.

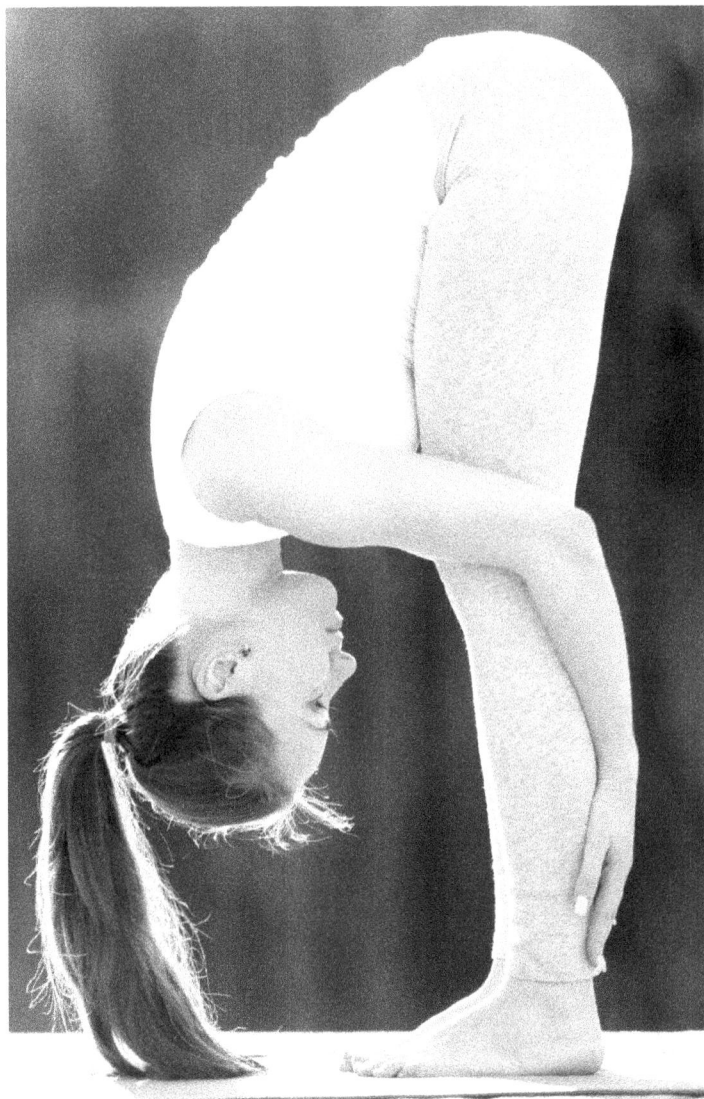

Upward Facing Dog Pose (Urdhva Mukha Svanasana)

Upward Facing Dog Pose is one of the most commonly known, as well as Downward Dog Pose, and recognized yoga pose due to its many benefits and healing uses. Similar to the Cobra Pose, it is thought of as one of the simplest of the back-bending poses and is implemented during the traditional Sun Salutation sequence.

How to Do

Lie face down on the floor. Stretch your legs back, with the tops of your feet on the floor. Bend your elbows and stretch your palms on the floor at the side of your waist so that your forearms are somewhat erect to the floor.

Breathe in and press your inner hands firmly into the floor and somewhat back, similar to trying to push yourself forward along the floor. Then at the same time, straighten your arms and lift your torso up and your legs a few inches off the floor on an intake breath. Keep the thighs firm and somewhat turned inward, the arms firm and turned out so the elbow creases face forward.

Press your tailbone toward your pubis and lift pubis toward your navel. Contract the hip positions. Stiffen but do not totally harden the buttocks.

Steady your shoulder blades against the back and puff the side ribs forward. Lift through the top of the sternum but make an effort not to push the front ribs forward. It will prompt the lower back to tighten. You will at that point look forward or you can angle your head towards the back slightly, remembering to take care not to constrict the back of your neck and the tightening of your throat.

Even though Upward Facing Dog Pose is one position used in the traditional Sun Salutation sequence, you can correspondingly practice this pose independently, maintaining the pose fifteen to thirty seconds, inhaling slowly. Release back to the floor or lift into the Downward Facing Dog pose along with an exhalation.

Benefits

Upward Facing Dog helps open the chest and strengthens the whole body and aligns the spine and invigorates nervous system and the kidneys.

Tips

Performing Upward Facing Dog will elongate and strengthen your whole body. You can use it as a backbend by itself, or as a transition for even deeper backbends.

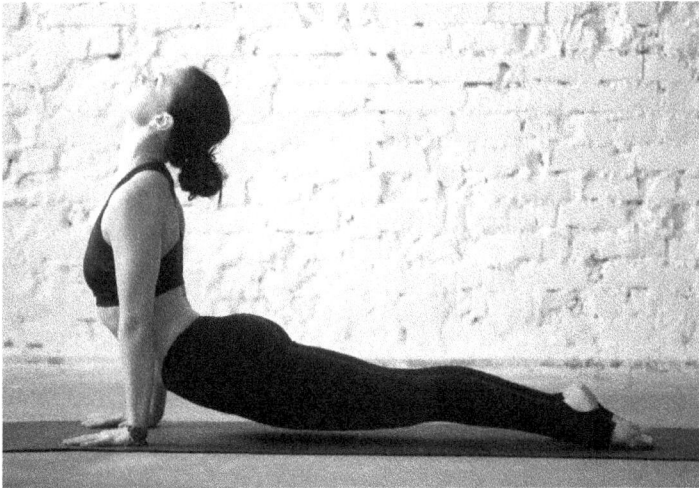

Downward Facing Dog Pose (Adho Mukha Svanasana)

Downward Facing Dog Pose is one of the traditional Sun Salutation sequences poses. It's also an excellent yoga asana all on its own.

How to Do

Begin with your hands and knees in a tabletop position. Make sure your shoulders are aligned above your wrists and your hips are aligned above your knees. Come to a flat back by lengthening the spine. Place your head and neck in a non-aligned position, staring down in the direction of the floor.

Breathe out and raise your knees away from the floor. At the start, keep your knees slightly bent and your heels lifted away from the floor. Lengthen your tailbone positioned from the back of your pelvis and press it slightly toward the pubis. Alongside this tension, raise the resting bones in the direction of the ceiling, and from your inner ankles pull the inner legs up into the groin.

Followed by letting your breath out, push your top thighs back and extend your heels against or down toward the floor. Making sure that you do not lock them, straighten your knees and steady your outer thighs, rolling the upper thighs inward slightly, narrowing the front of the pelvis.

Firming the outer arms, press the bottoms of your index fingers assertively into the floor. From these two points, lift alongside the inside of your arms from the wrists to the tops of the shoulders. Firm your shoulder blades against your back then widen them and draw them toward the tailbone. Keep your head between your upper arms; not allowing it to simply hang.

Continue in this pose somewhere between one to three minutes. Afterward, bend your knees to the floor with a breath and repose in the Child's Pose.

Benefits

Downward Facing Dog pose can help decrease back pain through strengthening the whole back and shoulder girdle. It aids in stronger hands, wrists, the Achilles tendon, low-back, hamstrings, and calves, as well as increasing the full-body circulation. Elongates your shoulders and shoulder blade area. Decrease in tension and headaches by elongating the cervical spine and neck and relaxing the head. It can also lessen anxiety and expand your respiration

Tips

You can alleviate the burden on your wrists by employing a block beneath your palms or you can be capable of completing the pose upon your elbows. By lifting your hands on blocks or the seat of a chair, you can help to release and open your shoulders.

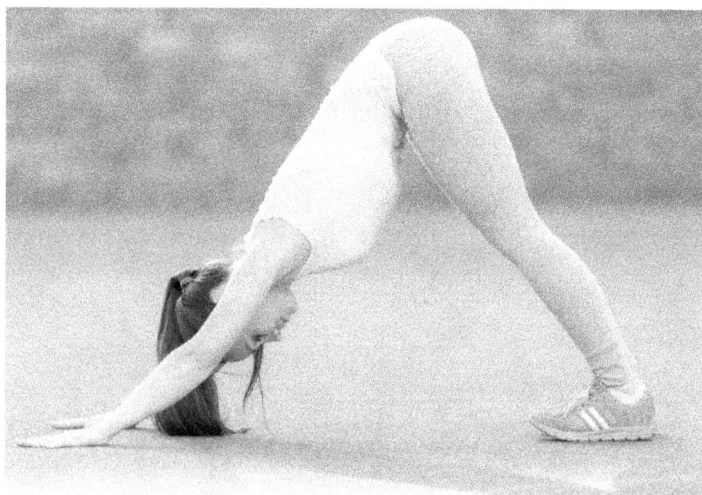

Handstand Pose (Adho Mukha Vrksasana)

The Handstand Pose is an advanced inversion and arm balance. The key powers of the handstand are to promote stability and strengthen the shoulders, arms, wrists, and the core. It is most frequently, to begin with practiced alongside a wall for safety and support. The Handstand is a pose that calls for caution and patience, but it is a worthwhile pose that increases focus and relieves stress.

How to Do

Start by moving yourself into Downward Facing Dog, positioning yourself two to five inches from the wall, but if you are a more experienced practitioner, you may feel comfortable without having a wall near. Your palms should be placed shoulder width apart, with your fingers facing forward, and your legs and spine should be nice and straight to create an inverted V shape. Be sure you ground your Downward Facing Dog before going forward. Progressing into the handstand is perhaps the most daunting part of this position, so creating a solid starting base is important.

As soon as you're prepared to move on, walk your feet closer to your palms. Fight the desire to move your head in closer to the wall. Keep your trunk in the same position, drawing it aside from the wall as you step forward. Don't bring in your feet in so close you become wobbly, but just enough you feel your hands create a strong base to the floor.

Bring one foot in closer, inclining the knee. This foot will be the one that helps launch you into the handstand position, so try out which one you are comfortable with. Hold your other leg stretched and active, but move your weight to the foot on your bowed leg. Lifting your extended leg to move your toes off the floor, hop a few times to ready yourself for the handstand. Swing your extended leg straight up, applying your bent leg to trigger the launch, before sweeping and spreading the bent leg. Legs have to be extended and jointly, soles of the feet in the direction of the ceiling. Work your core belly muscles to help raise your hips directly above your head and shoulders. Almost certainly, you cannot keep both legs up the initial few times you try to kick your legs up. Perhaps not at present, but if you persist to hop and kick both your legs up like this, you will move into the full handstand.

After you get both of your legs up into the complete handstand, commence by working to maintain the pose for ten to fifteen seconds, drawing the strong, measured breaths, until you can handle up to an entire sixty seconds. When moving out of the posture, work to swing both legs down, one after another, without flexing the spine or legs. This will aid in preventing you from transferring your weight onto your shoulders and neck.

Benefits

Expand your chest, strengthens the shoulders, arms, and wrists. Improves your balance and relieves stress.

Tips

Your grounded foot will lift easily when your weight is more forward of your wrists than behind them. Use your inhales to rock your weight forward, pull your belly in and hips up, and lift onto the ends of your standing toes until they lift themselves up. Once you're up, keep your balance by picking a point on the ground and keeping your eyes focused there.

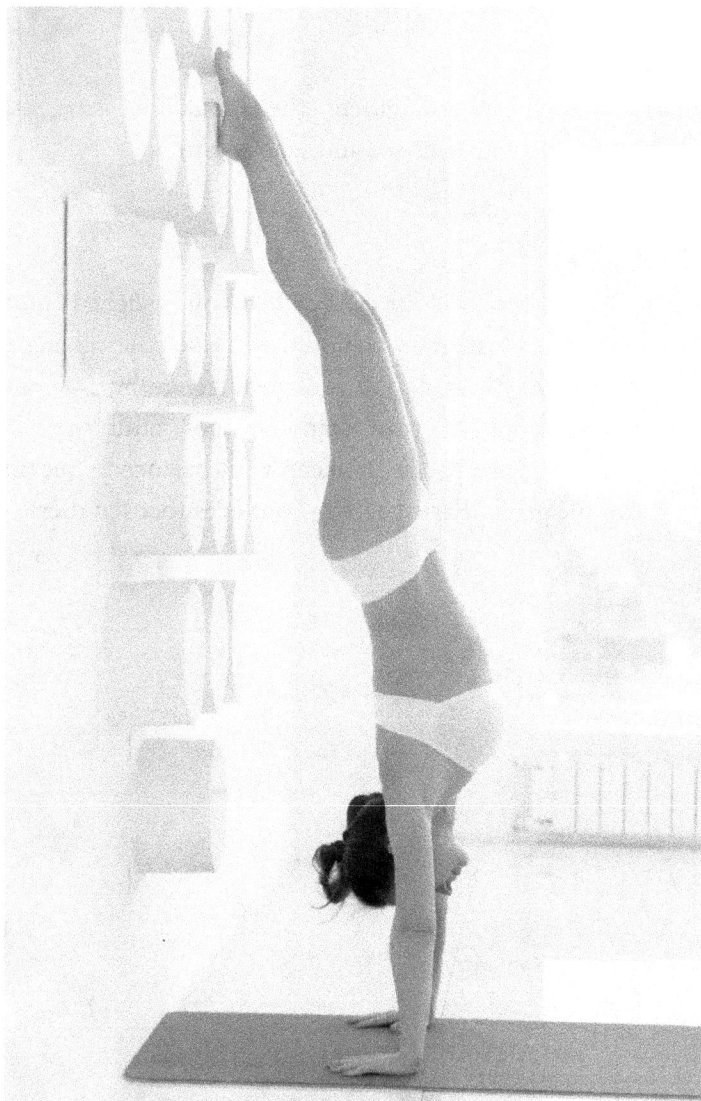

Child's Pose (Balasana)

The Child's Pose is a popular beginner's yoga posture. It is generally utilized as a resting position in among more difficult poses throughout a yoga practice.

How to Do

Come to all fours (Table Pose) exhale and lower your hips to your heels and forehead to the floor. Kneeling on the floor, bring your big toes together and sit on your heels, then separate your knees about as far as your hips.

Your arms can be above your head with your palms on the floor. Your palms can be flat or fisted with them stacked under your forehead, or your arms can be at the sides of your body with your palms up.

The Child's Pose is a resting pose. Remain in this position anywhere from thirty seconds to a few minutes. Beginners can also use this pose to get a feel of a deep forward bend. To come up, first stretch your front torso, followed by an inhalation lift from your tailbone as it pushes down and into your pelvis.

Benefits

The Child's Pose aids to stretch your hips, thighs, and ankles at the same time it reduces stress and fatigue. It gradually relaxes the muscles on the front of your body while softly and reflexively elongates the muscles of the back of your torso.

As it centers, calm, and soothes your brain, the Child's Pose is said to be a beneficial posture for alleviating stress. When done with your head and torso braced, it can as well help relieve back and neck pain.

The Child's Pose soothes the body, mind, and spirit while stimulating your third eye. Gently stretching the lower back, the Child's Pose massages and tones your abdominal organs, and encourages digestion and elimination.

Tips

Before you relax completely, press your palms into the ground with your arms straight and elbows lifted. Push your hips firmly back toward your heels. Breathe deeply into your whole back, for an extra release in your back. Make use of this pose to rest in the middle of more challenging poses.

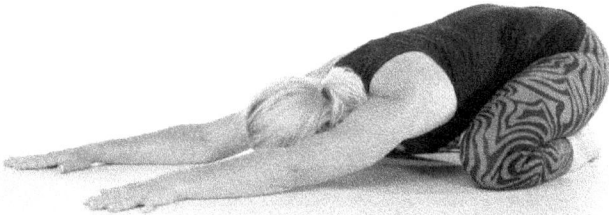

Corpse Pose (Shavasana)

The Corpse Pose is typically performed at the end of a yoga sequence. It can on the other hand be utilized at the start to calm your body before performing or in the midpoint of a sequence to rest. When applied at the conclusion of a yoga practice it is usually followed by a seated meditation phase to re-incorporate the body mind spirit back into the world.

How to Do

Lying on your back let your arms and legs drop open. With your arms at about forty five degrees from the side of your body, make sure you are comfortable and warm. With your eyes closed begin with slow deep breaths through the nose.

Allowing your entire body to become soft and heavy, let it relax onto the floor. As your body relaxes, feel your full body expanding and decreasing with each breath. Glance over your body from your toes to the top of your head, inspecting for any tension, stiffness or tightened muscles. Intentionally let go and relax any spots that you may find. Sway or shake those parts of your body from side to side to boost further release.

Let go of all control of your breath, your mind, and your body. Allow your body to move deeper and further into a state of complete relaxation. Remain in the Corpse Pose for five to fifteen minutes.

To release the Corpse Pose gradually deepen your breath, wriggle your fingers and toes, bring your arms over your head and stretch your entire body, breathing out, bend your knees into your chest, then roll over to one side going into the fetal position. Once you are ready, slowly inhaling, rising up into a seated position.

Benefits

The Corpse Pose allows your body and mind the time to sort out what has occurred during a yoga session. To most individuals, no yoga session is finished without this final pose. Your body needs this time to comprehend the new information it has received during the practice of yoga. Even though the Corpse Pose is a resting pose, you are not going to sleep.

Tips

Simply, relax. Follow your breathing without striving to control it. Observe what's taking place in your body. Gather your thoughts as they come along and let them go.

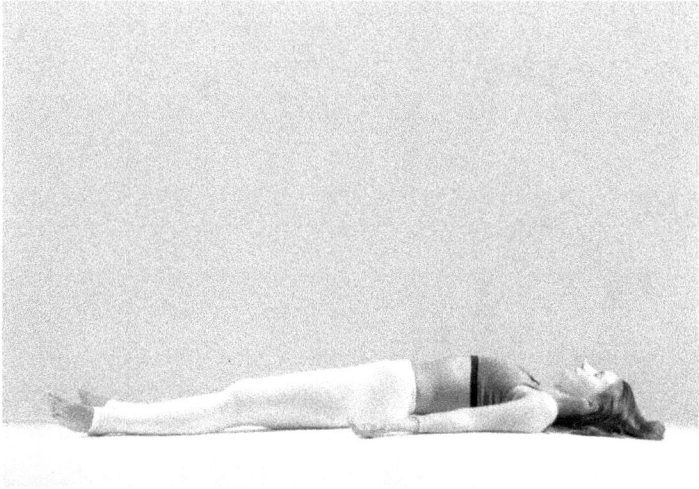

Constructing a Yoga Sequence

Here are a few points to keep in mind how to construct a yoga sequence. You are not at a studio, paying to be there. You do not have to exercise for over an hour. Begin with 5-10 minutes. Notice how you feel by the end of this time. If you feel as if you can do more, go ahead. If no, end your routine there.

Start with 5-10 minutes. By the conclusion of that time, notice how you feel. Do you desire to resume? If yes, continue for an extra five minutes and then check in with yourself once more. If not, close your workout.

The same as any physical journey, a yoga sequence has three clear parts.

Your opening or warm-up sequence

You don't want to jump into the main event tight and cold. This is where you move through and loosening up your major muscle groups as well as body parts

Your main sequence

Once you've warmed up, it's time for your main sequence. This component of your sequence is influenced by the goal of your routine. If it's an asymmetrical pose, keep in mind to do both sides and devote about the same time on each side.

The closing or cool down sequence

Now you've completed the principal portion of your yoga practice, it's time to cool down.

About The Author

Monique Joiner Siedlak is a writer, witch, and warrior on a mission to awaken people to their greatest potential through the power of storytelling infused with mysticism, modern paganism, and new age spirituality. At the young age of 12, she began rigorously studying the fascinating philosophy of Wicca. By the time she was 20, she was self-initiated into the craft, and hasn't looked back ever since. To this day, she has authored over 35 books pertaining to the magick and mysteries of life. Her most recent publication is book one of an Urban Paranormal series entitled "Jaeger Chronicles."

Originally from Long Island, New York, Monique is now a proud inhabitant of Northeast Florida; however, she considers herself to be a citizen of Mother Earth. When she doesn't have a book or pen in hand, she loves exploring new places and learning new things. And being the nature lover that she is, she considers herself to be an avid animal advocate.

To find out more about Monique Joiner Siedlak artistically, spiritually, and personally, feel free to visit her official website, www.mojosiedlak.com.

Other Books by Monique Joiner Siedlak

Mojo's Wiccan Series

Wiccan Basics

Candle Magick

Wiccan Spells

Love Spells

Abundance Spells

Hoodoo

Herb Magick

Seven African Powers: The Orishas

Moon Magick

Cooking for the Orishas

Creating Your Own Spells

Body Mind and Soul Series

Creative Visualization

Astral Projection for Beginners

Meditation for Beginners

Reiki for Beginners

Thorne Witch Series

The Phoenix

Beautiful You Series

Creating Your Own Body Butter

Creating Your Own Body Scrub

Creating Your Own Body Spray

Mojo's Self-Improvement Series

Manifesting With the Law of Attraction

Stress Management

Jaeger Chronicles

Glen Cove

Connect With Me!

I really appreciate you reading my book! Please leave a review and let me know your thoughts. Here are the social media locations you can find me at:

Like my **Facebook Page**: www.facebook.com/mojosiedlak

Follow me on **Twitter**: www.twitter.com/mojosiedlak

Follow me on **Instagram**: www.instagram.com/mojosiedlak

Follow me on **Bookbub**: http://bit.ly/2KEMkqt

Sign up to my **Email List** at www.mojosiedlak.com and receive a free book!

If you enjoyed this book or found it useful I'd be very grateful if you'd post a short review on at your retailer. Your support really does make a difference and I read all the reviews personally so I can get your feedback and make this as well as the next book even better.